WALKING WITH ABRAHAM & SARAH

Six weeks of devotions for body and spirit

Susan Martins Miller

Healthy Living
for Church and Home
❖RESOURCES FROM CHURCH HEALTH

Founded in 1987, Church Health is a charitably funded, faith-based, not-for-profit organization with a mission to *reclaim the church's biblical commitment to care for our bodies and our spirits.* Church Health provides comprehensive, high-quality, affordable health care to uninsured and underserved individuals and their families and gives people tools to live healthier lives. With the generous support of volunteer providers, the faith community, donors and community partners, we work tirelessly to improve health and well-being so that people can experience the full richness of life. For more information visit www.ChurchHealth.org.

Walking with Abraham and Sarah: Six Weeks of Devotions for Body and Spirit
© 2013, 2020 Church Health Center, Inc. Memphis, TN

ISBN: 978-1-62144-068-0

Healthy Living for Church and Home brings you practical tools and insights to help you faithfully create habits to honor God and know fullness of life.

Walking with Abraham and Sarah is part of the Ways to Wellness series, which also includes *Walking with Jesus* and *Walking with Paul.*

Written by Susan Martins Miller.

Cover and interior design by Lizy Heard.

Our Mission

CHURCH HEALTH is a faith-based organization. Each day, we stand ready to care for people who are hurting but live within a health care system that has left them behind. Our neighbors come seeking help, yet what they find is much deeper and more healing. They discover hope for a better life.

The Bible calls us to follow Jesus, which means helping people farther along the path to knowing God by showing God's love through our actions to heal both body and spirit. Because the Bible guides our understanding of God's love as well as God's calling for us, we share the Bible's commitment to bring wellness and hope to people of all circumstances.

We know from history that Christians have always cared for the underserved, both in body and spirit. Jesus asks us to care about what he cares about—wellness and wholeness of all people. Healing that flows through personal care, preventive activities, medical methods, and health technology announce that God is present among us.

God invites us to participate in the overarching story of God's love in the world. The commitment to care for bodies and spirits belongs to the church—both locally and worldwide—because the church belongs to Jesus.

In Memphis, Tennessee, Church Health provides clinical services to uninsured and underserved individuals in the areas of medical, dental, optometry, physical rehabilitation, and behavioral health, along with wellness services in nutrition, life health coaching, child well-being, and disease prevention. Our funding comes from charitable sources, and hundreds of volunteers augment our staff to care for thousands of patients. Beyond Memphis, we reach across the country and around the globe with a ministry of faith community nurses and publications for healthy living.

Your purchase and use of this publication shares in our mission to care for bodies and spirits in a way that shows the love and hope of Jesus on the road to living in healthier ways that honor God's love for us.

For more information visit www.ChurchHealth.org.

Introduction

WELCOME TO *Walking with Abraham and Sarah*, a six-week experience designed to help you make small changes and simple lifestyle improvements in your health and to grow in faith by accomplishing three simple goals:

1. Add 2,000 more steps a day to your activity level.
2. Add 3 servings of vegetables to your daily meals.
3. Add 3 glasses of water (a total of 24 ounces) each day to your daily fluids.

An inspiring devotional dimension reminds you of the connection between health in body and spirit. As you work on physical health goals, daily Scripture readings and meditations help you follow the routes that Jesus walked and nurture your spirit as well.

GETTING STARTED

You may choose to complete *Walking with Abraham and Sarah* on your own, with a friend or two, or as part of a program organized through your congregation or community group.

To get started, you'll want to know the baseline for how many steps you take in a typical day, how many servings of vegetables you eat, and how much water you drink.

1. **STEPS.** If you don't have a good idea of the number of steps you take in a day, plan on using the first three days to maintain a normal activity level, but keep track of your steps. You can use a pedometer or convert minutes of activity into steps using the Activity Conversion Chart on page 11. Average your number of steps during the first three days to set your baseline.

   For instance, Tom walked, 5,050 steps on Monday, 4,123 steps on Tuesday, and 6,233 steps on Wednesday. This adds up to a total of 15,406 steps. He'll divide the number by three to get an average of 5,135 steps per day. This is Tom's baseline.

   Then the goal will be to increase the daily steps by 2,000. If your baseline is about 5,000 steps, then you'll aim for 7,000 steps each day. If your baseline is 3,000 steps, then you'll aim for 5,000. You won't be comparing yourself to anyone else—only where you've been and where you want to go.

2. **VEGETABLES.** For three days, record how many servings of vegetables you eat. One serving is one-half cup cooked or one cup raw vegetables. Find your average for the three days. That is your baseline. The goal is to add three more. If your average is two servings, aim for five. If your average is four, aim for seven.

3. **WATER.** For three days, keep track of how many times you drink at least eight ounces of water. Find your average for the three days. That is your baseline. Adding three glasses per day (a total of 24 ounces) can be as simple as drinking eight ounces (one cup) of water at each of three meals.

— MY PERSONAL RECORD —

Program Start Date: ....

My baseline steps ....   My steps goal ....

My baseline vegetables ....   My vegetables goal ....

My baseline water ....   My water goal ....

BENEFITS OF *WALKING WITH ABRAHAM AND SARAH*

The eating and physical activity patterns of the majority of Americans have made us the most overweight nation in the world. More than 60 percent of American adults do not get the recommended 30 minutes of physical activity in a day, and 25 percent are not physically active at all. Nearly two-thirds of adults are overweight, with the average person gaining one or two pounds each year.

This six-week experience will:
- Inspire individuals, groups of friends, or whole congregations to engage in fun, simple ways to become more active and eat more healthfully (and move toward a healthy weight as needed).
- Create a supportive network for changes in individual and congregational behavior.
- Encourage everyone who participates to use their gifts to live a healthy life.

It's all about energy balance! We can manage weight gain by creating a healthier balance between the amount of energy burned and the types and amount of food consumed throughout a normal day. Small changes, such as the three goals in this program, can make a difference without creating a sense of impossibility or failure. The key is reasonable and achievable goals. Big change doesn't happen all at once, but one step at a time—literally.

TOOLS IN THIS BOOK

You'll want to keep a Bible handy as you read each day's meditation. Many Bibles include maps that may help you identify locations mentioned in the passages you read. A simple **MAP**, such as on the back cover, gives you an appreciation for the places and distances Jesus traveled.

Each day's reading page also includes a **DAILY HEALTH JOURNAL** where you can record your number of steps for that day and check off whether you met the goals of adding 2,000 steps, 3 servings of vegetables, and 3 glasses of water. At the end of each week, transfer your checkmarks to a summary chart and see how you did for the week overall.

In addition to the daily meditations, each day provides a new **HEALTH TIP** to share health information or encourage you to incorporate what you already know into your daily routines.

At the close of this introductory material, you'll also find **TIPS FOR ADDING STEPS TO YOUR DAY** and an **ACTIVITY CONVERSION CHART** to help you calculate how other physical activity equates to added steps. Bicycling, gardening, yoga, rollerblading—it all counts toward walking. If you would also like to trim calories, a bonus goal, you'll find **TIPS FOR CUTTING 100 CALORIES**.

To begin your six weeks of walking, consider using the Self-assessment on page 13 that invites you to record you baseline habits and attitudes. Share this with a friend or turn it in to a project coordinator if you are part of a congregational program. At the end of six weeks, you'll have another opportunity to answer similar questions, evaluate your progress, and set new goals.

WALKING WITH ABRAHAM AND SARAH IN A GROUP

Many features of *Walking with Abraham and Sarah* are for individual use—keeping the Daily Health Journal, setting personal goals, and seeking spiritual inspiration in the daily reflections you can read at any time of the day. This doesn't mean you have to be on your own. You might be a leader looking for a simple program to use in your congregation to encourage healthy habits, or you might be someone who wants to gather a few friends for a shared path for six weeks of accountability as you all set reasonable goals and support each other in reaching them. Whether a handful of friends or a congregation-wide program, *Walking with Abraham and Sarah* works well for group use.

Here are a few tips.

1. **ORDER COPIES IN ADVANCE.** If you're reading this copy of *Walking with Abraham and Sarah* and want to organize a group, make it easy by ordering copies for your group at one time. Make sure everyone has a copy before the start of the six-week period.

2. **HOLD A BRIEF LAUNCH MEETING.** This doesn't have to be long or involved. The purpose is to draw attention to the tools in the book and agree together how you want to use them in your group. This gets everyone on the same page so that as you support each other over the six-week period, everyone speaks the same language. Will you share the pre- and post-assessments?

What do you think will be the best ways you'll want to add steps or cut calories from the tips lists provided? How often will you connect with each other?

3. **PLAN WAYS TO TOUCH BASE.** Knowing how to support each other will be important. Some ideas are:
- Meet for a few minutes during the coffee time or adult Sunday school hour on Sunday mornings and talk about successes and challenges of the week. Share which reflections encouraged you the most. Pray for one another.
- Set up a closed Facebook group and post daily questions for members to respond to about how they're doing on their health journeys. Consider ways to tie questions to the daily reflections or health tips.
- Use a group e-mail, text message, or Messenger process for frequent private contact with words of encouragement, tips, and brief prayers.
- Plan times when members of the group can physically walk together and share their successes and challenges and get some steps in at the same time. The whole group doesn't have to walk together. This could be a time for two to four people to meet up according to schedules or locations.

4. **SHARE A CLOSING MEAL.** At the end of six weeks, share a healthy meal. Invite participants who shared the walking journey to bring healthy dishes that reflect ways they changed their eating during the six weeks. There might be some recipe swapping!

Each new healthy habit becomes a foundation for the next one. One of the best ways to celebrate progress is to know your starting point and be able to look back after six weeks and see changes. No change for the better is too small to celebrate.

TIPS FOR ADDING STEPS TO YOUR DAY
Making simple choices to add steps throughout your day will result in an added 2,000 steps before you know it. Try some of these ideas.

Choose the stairs instead of the elevator.
Park in the back row of the parking lot.
Mow the lawn with a walking mower.
Walk with a friend during your lunch break.
Pace around the house while talking on the phone.
Instead of e-mailing or calling a coworker, walk down the hall and have a face-to-face interaction.
Make several trips and up and down the stairs when doing laundry and household chores.
Pass the drive-thru and walk into the restaurant or bank.
Tour a museum, zoo, or nature preserve.
Volunteer to walk dogs for an animal shelter.
Walk to yard sales to shop for bargains.
Circle around the block once before bringing in the mail.
Walk on short errands, such as a nearby store, post office, or dry cleaners.
Go window shopping at the mall.
Meet a friend for lunch at a restaurant you can walk to.
Play a round of golf but pass on the golf cart.

TIPS FOR CUTTING 100 CALORIES

Small changes in food preparation and portion size can quickly add up and have a dramatic impact on your health. Each one of these options will allow you to trim 100 calories out of your daily intake and meet your daily goal.

Select skim, one percent or two percent milk instead of whole milk.

Use a small glass for juice and a small bowl for cereal.

Use cooking spray in place of butter or margarine.

Put lettuce, tomato, onions, and pickles on your burger or sandwich instead of cheese.

Prepare tuna or chicken salad with fat-free or light mayonnaise.

Select soft corn tortillas instead of hard shell tortillas.

Replace a can of soda with mineral water.

Enjoy your salad without the croutons.

Leave three or four bites on your plate.

Use a fat-free, light, or reduced-fat cheese, sour cream, or salad dressing in place of regular.

Limit meat portions to three or four ounces—the size of a deck of cards.

Steam vegetables rather than frying with butter.

Add 1/4 less cheese to spaghetti and lasagna. Customize the dish with fresh seasonal vegetables.

Bake, broil, or grill chicken instead of frying.

Share one serving of dessert with a friend.

Substitute applesauce for vegetable oil when baking.

Choose 100 percent juice over juice cocktails and fruit punch.

Skip super-sized portions.

Choose a side salad or steamed vegetables instead of fries, pasta, or onion rings.

Dip your fork in salad dressing instead of pouring dressing over the salad.

Cut out one tablespoon of butter or oil from a recipe.

Use two egg whites in place of one whole egg.

ACTIVITY CONVERSION CHART

If you engage in physical activities other than walking, you can convert minutes of activity to steps for credit toward adding 2,000 steps per day to your usual routine.

Activity	Steps per Minute
Aerobics (low-impact)	125
Aerobics (moderate)	153
Aerobics (water)	100
Basketball	100
Bicycling (leisurely)	100
Bicycling (moderate)	200
Bicycling (stationary)	181
Cross country skiing	114
Dancing (all types)	133
Elliptical machine	203
Football	133
Gardening	73
Golf (walking)	100
Jogging (12 minutes per mile)	232
Hopping	51
Painting	78
Pilates	92
Racquetball	138
Resistance training	74
Rollerblading	200
Rowing (leisurely)	74
Rowing (moderate)	153
Running (10 minutes per mile)	290
Running (7.5 minutes per mile)	391
Scrubbing floors	92
Soccer	144
Stair climbing (down)	72

Continued on page 12.

Continued from page 11.

Activity	Steps per Minute
Stair climbing (up)	205
Stretching	6
Swimming	200
Tai chi	8
Tennis	200
Volleyball	90
Walking	125
Washing car	72
Waterskiing	136
Weight lifting	100
Yoga	50

— Self-assessment —

If you are using **Walking with Abraham and Sarah** *as part of a group or congregation, answer these questions before you begin and consider sharing your answers with the project coordinator or friends in your group.*

Name: ....

Congregation or Community Organization: ....

....

1. How many days a week do you engage in some type of mild to moderate physical activity (walking slowly, gardening, housework, window shopping, and so on)? Days per week ....

2. How many days a week do you engage in some type of moderate to vigorous physical activity (brisk walking, running, riding a bike, dancing, playing a sport and so on)? Days per week ....

3. Which answer best describes how you feel about the following?

	I have no plans to	I plan to in the future	I plan to immediately	I have been doing so for *fewer* than six months	I have been doing so for *more* than six months
Increasing physical activity					
Improving nutrition					

4. To what degree do you feel that your physical health and spiritual health are connected?

○ Not at all   ○ Quite a bit
○ A little bit   ○ Extremely
○ Moderately

CUT HERE

Begin Your Journey
HERE

Take Us to Tomorrow

GENESIS 12:1-3

*"Go from your country and your kindred and your
father's house to the land that I will show you."*
—Genesis 12:1

GOD CALLED ABRAM to leave his country in an act of faith, not knowing where he was going.

Abram (as Abraham was known at this stage in his life) had a place where he belonged, where he knew the patterns of daily life and where his extended family knew him. Life may not have been perfect, but Abram would have known what to expect from daily routine. All this he was to exchange for a new journey with God. Note that God did not simply say, "Get out of here and figure it out yourself." Rather, God's message in Genesis 12:1-3 was that God would be present in this unknown future and even would bless him. Abram was not being evicted with nowhere to go. God would show him what was ahead. The promises God makes in these verses reiterate that the journey will enrich Abram, his family, and people Abram did not even know. One encounter with God after another lay ahead for Abram even when his faith faltered. Something truly great would come from saying "Yes" to this call.

At the start of six weeks of walking with Abraham and Sarah, we hear the call to leave behind patterns that are comfortable—even if they are not good for us—and walk toward the well-being and blessing God has in store for us. And we are not alone on this strange journey any more than Abram was.

HEALTH TIP

When we worry about an unknown future we often imagine the worst. This causes stress, which can affect health in negative ways. Certain activities, such as journaling, yoga, religious practices, and even laughter have been found to lower stress. By engaging in stress-reducing activities, we can keep our bodies from going into chronic stress mode and support our own health and wellness. Identify one source of stress in your life and one way to address the stress.

— DAILY HEALTH JOURNAL —

Number of steps........................ ○ Add 3 servings of vegetables
○ Add 2,000 steps ○ Add 3 glasses of water

The Gift of Aging

GENESIS 12:4

Abram was seventy-five years
old when he departed from Haran.
—Genesis 12:4

BY OUR STANDARDS TODAY, Abram was not a young man when he heard the call of God and answered. Though we do not know how much time was required to ready his household for this change, the writer of Genesis leaves no gap in the storytelling. God told Abram to go, and he went. Abram did not say, "I'm too old for this" or "It's too late for me" or "It's too late to change now because the damage is already done" or any of the other excuses we might pull out when confronted with the call to make significant changes in our lives. He didn't argue that packing up and moving to a new land, literally or metaphorically, was something for the young folks. God could have called a younger person, but he called someone who was 75 as an example of how to live through changing times. As we age, Abram's story is a good reminder that no matter how old we are, the future still lies ahead, and God asks us to be open to where God might lead.

Anyone who has read the story of Abram before knows that departing from Haran was just the beginning of his faith adventures. Our decisions to make even small changes in health habits are also just the beginning of our adventures. God, our redeemer, calls us to wellness in both body and spirit, and an openness to being made new is just the beginning.

HEALTH TIP

What can we do to keep ourselves healthy even as we grow older? What lifestyle choices will allow us to continue to proclaim God's message and do God's work for many years to come? Some commonly accepted ways to maintain good health and energy as we age are to keep our weight in an acceptable range, exercise regularly, don't smoke, and eat a healthy diet. These sensible actions are all part and parcel of our mission to be faithful to God's call.

— DAILY HEALTH JOURNAL —

Number of steps............................   O Add 3 servings of vegetables

O Add 2,000 steps   O Add 3 glasses of water

Altars in the Landscape

GENESIS 12:5-7

So he built an altar to the LORD,
who had appeared to him.
—**Genesis 12:7**

ABRAM'S JOURNEY WAS NO SMALL undertaking. He didn't just grab a backpack and a walking stick, hoping to pick up a map along the way. His wife, Sarai, and nephew, Lot, who were his close relatives, traveled with him. Even more, he took his entire household—servants and others whom Abram was responsible for. He made appropriate plans for a successful journey and welcomed others to travel with him.

Abram traveled a considerable distance, venturing into a foreign land and arriving at Shechem, a significant city in Canaan. There he heard from God again with encouraging words for the future. This very land, which must have felt so unfamiliar, would one day belong to his family.

Abram responded to God's encouragement by building an altar to mark the experience. As Abram's story unfolds, we see that he often built an altar in significant places on his journey with God.

Our health journeys may take us to unfamiliar places. We learn from Abram to open ourselves to how new places—and new habits—can become where we live and flourish. None of us travels in isolation. Choices we make about our health can encourage or discourage others in their own health journeys. As we travel through life, how many altars dot the landscape? How often have we taken the time to build into our lives sacred places and sacred moments?

HEALTH TIP

Holistic health means paying attention to our spirits as well as our bodies. We can encourage our spirits by periodically pausing to honor those have helped us along the way. Taking time to reflect on and thank those who help us on the health journey, such as walking partners, exercise instructors, and nutrition advisors, will spur us on to continued enthusiasm for the call to unexpected places.

— DAILY HEALTH JOURNAL —

Number of steps.............................   ○ Add 3 servings of vegetables
○ Add 2,000 steps   ○ Add 3 glasses of water

Patience with Stages

GENESIS 12:8–9

*And Abram journeyed on
by stages toward the Negeb.*
—Genesis 12:9

ABRAM AND SARAI CONTINUE their pilgrimage into this strange land. Their possessions—and Lot's—included considerable livestock, so they may have kept traveling south in search of sufficient land to support the household. They traveled past Bethel, a place where their grandson Jacob would one day have his own encounter with God (Genesis 28:10–22), though at the time they did not imagine he would ever exist. Once again Abram paused to build an altar and call on the name of God for the journey ahead.

Abram and Sarai traveled south in stages, not expecting to instantly or easily be at the end of the journey but to rely on God's strength in the journeying. The Negeb was an arid wilderness of the region Abram's descendants, many generations later, would call Judah. Caravans of donkeys and camels laden with goods from around the known world traveled through this cultural crossroads on the way to the prosperous markets of Egypt.

Did Abram and Sarai think their journey had come to an end? Probably not. But it seemed that the Negeb, even with its desert features, was the next stage of their obedience journey, and they did not shy away from it. In the same way, we should not expect quick fixes. Even poor health habits form over time, so reforming them takes time and stages as well.

HEALTH TIP

Sometimes the many nutrition facts and complex exercise routines can overwhelm the well-intentioned health pilgrim who is venturing into an unknown land that can seem like a wasteland. This can lead to procrastination and avoidance of needed steps forward. Nutrition and exercise do not have to be complicated. Begin simply. The most important thing is to begin! Then learn more and more by stages, not rushing too far ahead on the road to good health that you risk losing your way.

--- **DAILY HEALTH JOURNAL** ---

Number of steps...........................   O Add 3 servings of vegetables
O Add 2,000 steps   O Add 3 glasses of water

When Danger Looms
GENESIS 12:10-13

*So Abram went down to Egypt to reside there
as an alien, for the famine was severe in the land.*
—Genesis 12:10

FAMINE CHANGED EVERYTHING. The looming possibility of not having enough to eat shows a less secure side of Abram. Looking toward Egypt made sense because the Nile River's water supply was reliable and could be used to irrigate land and grow food. Abram left the land that God said would one day belong to his descendants because he needed to feed his household.

We get our first glimpse of Sarai in this part of the story. Although she was over 65 years old at the time, she was still regarded as beautiful, and Abram knew she would attract attention. They were traveling with an entourage of people and flocks and herds. They would not have been able to simply slip into Egypt, buy a supply of grain, and slip out. Sarai's beauty would be noticed, and if Pharaoh wanted to take her into his harem he would first have to dispose of her husband.

"Say you are my sister," Abram said to his wife, seeking to spare his own life. Under stress, Abram fell back on a technicality—Sarai was his *half*-sister, born of the same father—to justify his actions.

We don't have to think hard about how easily we justify some of our poor choices when it comes to health. A healthy habit is to step back and name the stress that makes us want to take the easy way out.

HEALTH TIP

God provides an abundance of naturally healthy food options. Try to select fresh fruits and vegetables in place of canned produced and processed snack foods. Following the current USDA guidelines will help you make nutritious choices and build variety into your eating habits. Planning in advance what you will eat throughout the day also will help you monitor portion size.

— DAILY HEALTH JOURNAL —

Number of steps.............................   ○ Add 3 servings of vegetables
○ Add 2,000 steps   ○ Add 3 glasses of water

Desperate Choices

GENESIS 12:14–20

So Pharaoh called Abram, and said,
"What is this you have done to me?"
—**Genesis 12:18**

ABRAM'S FEARS PROVED well founded. Sarai's beauty did attract notice, and she was taken into Pharaoh's household. Because of Sarai, Pharaoh's dealings with Abram were positive.

All that changed when plagues broke out in Pharaoh's house. Somehow the ruler put the pieces together and went straight back to Abram with the accusation that Abram was responsible for the suffering that had come to Pharaoh's house. In the end, Pharaoh discovered that while Abram had told some of the truth, he had kept back part of it to protect himself even if it meant putting his wife at risk.

With our twenty-first century culture and understanding of marriage and honor, we have a hard time reconciling Abram's actions. Perhaps the real question is how much of ourselves we see in Abram. Do we try to save our own skin? Do we try to work around the hard stuff? Do we put others at risk in order to get what we want?

Health is not only about nutrition and exercise for our bodies. It's also about relationships, emotions, and faith. Our deepest fears can stir up choices that are not good for us or for the people we care about.

HEALTH TIP

Do you find yourself overindulging in high-fat foods or alcohol just because you are in a social setting? If you cave into pressure—as Abram did—don't punish yourself for exercising poor judgment in a moment of stress. Instead, develop an action plan. Think of the barriers that prevent you from reaching health goals and build a plan not just to avoid them but to face them. If you get off track, allow yourself to start fresh.

— **DAILY HEALTH JOURNAL** —

Number of steps........................   ◯ Add 3 servings of vegetables
◯ Add 2,000 steps   ◯ Add 3 glasses of water

Along the Way
GENESIS 13:1-4

There Abram called on the name of the LORD.
—Genesis 13:4

AFTER THE DEBACLE IN EGYPT, Pharaoh sent Abram out of the country. Abram and Sarai, and their entire household, headed back to the Negeb wilderness. Genesis 13:2 tells us what we already suspected—that Abram was a wealthy man. But even with all his silver and gold, Abram had to journey through the wilderness toward wholeness. He returned to the place where Abram had built an altar (Genesis 12:8) and called on the name of the Lord. It was time to do this again and regain his spiritual bearings.

Sometimes when we find ourselves disappointed with our own choices, we need to go back to a time and place where we made a wise choice. Willpower is not the only strategy available to us. Like Abram, when we reset our spiritual bearings by tending to the ways we experience and express our faith, we are also taking an important step in managing the kinds of everyday experiences that trip us up and cause repercussions for our health.

No matter how many times we falter, God always offers a fresh start. Let's give ourselves grace to accept it.

HEALTH TIP

Hippocrates said, "A wise man should consider that health is the greatest of human blessings, and learn how by his own thought to derive benefits from his illness." Has recovery from an illness or surgery ever brought you back to your center and an awareness of what a gift good health is? These significant moments can be occasions for reaffirming commitment to a healthy lifestyle and awareness of God's wish for your continued wholeness.

— DAILY HEALTH JOURNAL —

Number of steps.................................   ⭘ Add 3 servings of vegetables
⭘ Add 2,000 steps   ⭘ Add 3 glasses of water

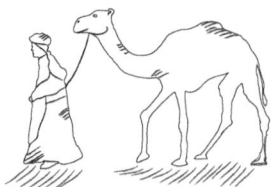

Week One in Review

THIS WEEK AS WE FOLLOWED the journey of Abraham and Sarah, we were struck with the magnitude of their faith. How many of us would pick up our lives at any ages—especially at 75—and move across the country without being certain of where were were going or why she would want to go there? Acting on trust, Abraham and Sarah journeyed across unfamiliar territory. They weren't perfect; they made mistakes. But they returned to their spiritual center and continued the journey.

Reflecting on the Scripture passages this week, perhaps you found yourself thinking through the stages of your own life's journey. The experiences of Abraham and Sarah help us realize that we do not need to rush ahead of God's call but rather proceed in stages through our lives while listening carefully for God's voice. There will be days when we struggle—even fail. But there will also be days when we succeed. We continue to trust God's provision for us and to live in gratitude for God's guidance.

Along with these reflections, include plenty of physical activity and foods that truly nourish your body. Taking the daily small steps that keep you on course will strengthen you not only physically but spiritually.

Transfer your daily steps in the space below. If you set a goal
for all three categories, put checkmarks in the boxes
where you reached your goal for each day.

Number of steps	Add 2,000 steps	Add 3 vegetables	Add 3 glasses of water
Day 1	O	O	O
Day 2	O	O	O
Day 3	O	O	O
Day 4	O	O	O
Day 5	O	O	O
Day 6	O	O	O
Day 7	O	O	O

People Matter
GENESIS 13:5-9

Then Abram said to Lot, "Let there be no strife between you and me."
—Genesis 13:8

REMEMBER, ABRAM AND LOT, with their household and considerable livestock, are in the Negeb, an arid region. Abram had become wealthy, and Lot was doing well also. Though a wilderness, the Negeb was not unpopulated. Canaanites and Perizzites already lived there, so newcomers Abram and Lot had limitations on the land they could use as pastures for the livestock. Then the land itself had limited water to support them.

Abram's animals seem to be clearly separated from Lot's, because their herdsmen began to quarrel about whose animals should have the better pastures. But Abram was not interested in fomenting a quarrel.

Abram saw not the limitations of the land but the abundance. He did not worry that if another person had enough, he would somehow not also have enough. Abram was simply confident that there was enough to go around and God would care for him as always. "Let there be no strife," he said as he offered Lot free choice of the land.

There was no reason for strife. How many situations do we find ourselves in where we feel pressure to take up sides, to declare who is right and who is wrong, when the truth is giving in to strife costs us a great deal in relationships and the meaning we find in our lives. We can take a lesson from Abram and think twice before fueling unnecessary and harmful strife when people are what matter most.

HEALTH TIP

Psychological health goes hand in hand with physical health. Having the skills to recognize and articulate our feelings and thoughts, and to respect another's feelings, is key in effective communicating, resolving conflict, and building relationships. Our circumstances may change and conflict may arise. Putting people first in the ways we respond to and resolve conflict will improve our health as well as theirs.

— DAILY HEALTH JOURNAL —

Number of steps........................   O Add 3 servings of vegetables
O Add 2,000 steps   O Add 3 glasses of water

Enough to Share

GENESIS 13:10-12

Abram settled in the land of Canaan,
while Lot settled among the cities of the Plain.
—**Genesis 13:12**

ABRAM TOOK THE INITIATIVE OF reconciliation by letting Lot choose the land he preferred without putting any conditions on the choice. Whatever Lot chose, Abram would be content with what remained.

Lot saw that land along the Jordan River would have sufficient irrigation, and he chose this and began his journey to the east.

We might think that Abram got the "leftover" land—what Lot had deemed as not good enough was somehow supposed to be good enough for his uncle. We might think that Lot went where he believed life would be easier and left his uncle to make do in a more difficult environment. We might even think that Lot made the selfish choice. But we would be reading our own attitudes into the story, because the passage tells us none of that.

Abram did not secretly hope that Lot would choose the more difficult land. He did not bear a grudge when Lot chose the water of the Jordan.

Sacrifice for the good of another is noble, but the greater lesson is that Abram followed through with a positive spirit about the outcome. Holding grudges causes stress, stirs up negative choices in our words and behavior, and cuts us off from people who enrich our lives. It's bad for our health!

HEALTH TIP

Our attitude toward illness and health, or toward challenging circumstances, can spell the difference between acceptance and fulfillment. Many times we need to change our outlook before we are able to change our behavior. Take time today to review some of the attitudes that you might want to let go of before you can follow through on the choices that will lead to better health in body and spirit.

— DAILY HEALTH JOURNAL —

Number of steps............................   O Add 3 servings of vegetables

O Add 2,000 steps   O Add 3 glasses of water

Lift Up Your Eyes

GENESIS 13:14-18

*"Raise your eyes now, and look
from the place where you are."*
—**Genesis 13:14**

WHEN ABRAM AND SARAI OBEYED God's call to a map-free journey, Lot went with them. Now Lot and Abram have separated so that each would have land enough for the prosperity they enjoyed. This is not to say they never expected to see one another again, but it certainly would have been an adjustment. Changes in the stages of our lives often are good times to take stock of where we are and where we're headed.

This is what God asked Abram to do now. "Raise your eyes now, and look from the place where you are." God promised to give all the land Abram could see to him and his offspring. And Abram had no children!

Imagine the expanse of land God offered—everything Abram could see in every direction. Sometimes, when we feel stuck, we have a hard time raising our eyes to look beyond immediate circumstances. This holds true for major decisions or simple health choices that take us closer to our goals.

Then God asked Abram to do one more thing: Rise up and walk through the land. Walking the land could have been either to inspect it or to symbolically claim it as the place he would live.

Raise your eyes from where you are on your health journey, which may feel dry and arid like the Negeb, and see what God wants to give you in the abundant life. Then start walking.

HEALTH TIP

Studies reveal that older adults who practice private religious activities, such as prayer, meditation, or reading the Bible, have a higher quality of life and illness recovery rate than those who do not. In fact, prayer and meditation can lead to a variety of health benefits. These include increased blood flow, decreased blood pressure, relaxed muscles, lower stress hormone levels, improved brain function, and more restful sleep.

— DAILY HEALTH JOURNAL —

Number of steps ....
- ○ Add 2,000 steps

- ○ Add 3 servings of vegetables
- ○ Add 3 glasses of water

Unexpected Sightings

GENESIS 14:11–20

*And King Melchizedek of Salem brought out bread
and wine; he was priest of God Most High.*
—Genesis 14:18

SOMETIME AFTER MOVING TO THE LAND he chose near Sodom and Gomorrah, Lot was caught in a war between regional kings and captured by an invading enemy. Someone escaped and went to tell Abram, who set off with a force of 318 trained soldiers, routed the enemy, and freed Lot. On his way home, he met met King Melchizedek of Salem (Jerusalem), a "priest of God Most High."

Melchizedek offered Abram both hospitality—bread and wine would have been an ordinary meal—and, more significant, a blessing in the name of God, whom they both worshiped.

We know nothing more about Melchizedek than what we learn in this chapter of Genesis and a summary of these events that appears in the New Testament book of Hebrews (7:1–3). He seems to come from nowhere and fade back into obscurity. But Abram recognized in him someone who knew the same God Abram knew and received his blessing with gratitude.

Until this point in Abram's story, we have not met anyone outside his household who worshiped God. Considering where Abram had just come from, the region of Sodom and Gomorrah known for deep wickedness, Abram could have been quite surprised to meet someone like Melchizedek. We meet servants of God in unexpected places if we open our hearts to recognize God's presence, and the blessing they offer may be just what we need to continue the journey to wholeness.

HEALTH TIP

One thing that has not changed between Abraham's time and ours is the benefit of shared meals. When families eat together, their relationships become stronger, the children tend to do better in school, food prepared at home may be more nutritious, and it's an opportunity to share spiritual traditions. All of these benefits improve health over a lifetime.

— DAILY HEALTH JOURNAL —

Number of steps............................   ○ Add 3 servings of vegetables

○ Add 2,000 steps   ○ Add 3 glasses of water

Counting the Stars
GENESIS 15:1-6

"Do not be afraid, Abram, I am your shield;
your reward shall be very great."
—Genesis 15:1

SEVERAL TIMES NOW GOD HAS PROMISED great blessing to Abram and Sarai through their offspring—but they are not getting any younger. Abram has heard these blessings with wonder, but when God came to him once again and said, "your reward shall be very great," Abram dared to push back.

What God promised looked impossible. Abram had no children. A slave born in his house was in line to inherit everything Abram had. Abram saw no solution. It was a nice idea but not likely to happen.

Health can be like that. We might think that God's goodness is not meant for us because we are ill or overweight or in chronic emotional pain—or childless. Some people believe that to ask questions of God is to lack faith. On the contrary, questions can express our desire to learn and understand God's movement in, and purpose for, our lives. Questions are one way that God knows we're paying attention!

God answered Abram's questions by repeating the promise once again, this time with the imagery of countless stars. "So shall your descendants be." And then God made a formal covenant with Abram (Genesis 15:7–11). The next time you think better health is impossible, go outside look at the stars. God's goodness is for you, just as it was for Abram.

HEALTH TIP

The Bible teaches about covenants established for God's people. A covenant is a binding agreement or promise. A covenant or a pledge is also a useful tool in making behavior changes. When you set a health goal, you make a pledge to yourself. Follow up in three or four weeks to review your progress. You may also want to make a promise with a friend to support each other in sustaining changes.

— DAILY HEALTH JOURNAL —

Number of steps.................   ○ Add 3 servings of vegetables
○ Add 2,000 steps   ○ Add 3 glasses of water

DAY 13

Through Terrifying Darkness

GENESIS 15:12–16

As the sun was going down, a deep sleep fell upon Abram,
and a deep and terrifying darkness descended upon him.
—**Genesis 15:12**

TO GIVE ABRAM THE ASSURANCE of a formal covenant or agreement, God told him to cut in half a heifer, a goat, and a ram. A turtledove and a pigeon were also part of the arrangement when Abram laid out the pieces that symbolized the covenant (Genesis 15:7–11). We can well imagine why Abram was tired!

We may be more confused why, after the greatness of God's promise, a "terrifying darkness" came to Abram. Though asleep, his encounter with God continued, and the message God gave was that the offspring God promised to give Abram, who would also inherit the land God gave Abram, would have dark seasons in their future. They would spend 400 years as slaves in a foreign land. This word from God came true generations later when Abram's great-grandsons and their families visited Egypt during a famine, as he had, and were eventually taken into slavery.

Coming off a promise of the stars, this would certainly be depressing news! Sometimes the way we feel about events in our lives, or the lives of those we love, is in contrast to events we have recently experienced. One way to be strong enough to bear the hard seasons is to be as healthy as possible in body and spirit during happier times. Healthy habits protect our mental outlook and our joy.

HEALTH TIP

During periods of depression or anxiety, exercise is a great way to release natural chemicals in your body to combat these low moods. Aim for 30 minutes of exercise three to five times a week to see significant improve of your symptoms, but if that is not possible, don't throw in the towel. As few as five to ten minutes of activity at a time can improve mood in the short term until you can get back on track.

— DAILY HEALTH JOURNAL —

Number of steps.............................   ○ Add 3 servings of vegetables

○ Add 2,000 steps   ○ Add 3 glasses of water

The Wall of Renewal

GENESIS 15:17–21

On that day the LORD made a covenant with Abram.
—**Genesis 15:18**

GOD PROMISED ABRAM descendants as numerous as the stars (Genesis 15:5), told Abram to prepare the physical form of a covenant by dividing the pieces of animals (Genesis 15:9), and told Abram of the oppression that lay ahead for his family (Genesis 15:13). By now it was dark, and the dominant image in this part of the story is a flaming torch that passed between the pieces of animals. In ancient times, when two parties made a covenant, they walked through the aisle created by the pieces of slaughtered animals, as if to say "This is what will happen to me if I do not keep my promise." The flaming torch is an image of God making a solemn promise by participating in the customary form of a binding covenant.

Abram did not walk between the animal pieces, which made this an unusual covenant. God did not say, "If you are good enough I will keep my promise" or "I will see if you keep your part before I keep mine." God assumed the burden of this promise and gave Abram a vision beyond the immediate circumstances—hope.

We sometimes think we have to clean up our act before we can ask for God's help or presence. But that is not the lesson from this story. Quite the opposite. God is present in our struggles and our joys. We do not walk the path to better health alone.

HEALTH TIP

God used a physical sign of fire to symbolize his commitment to Abram. You also can use something physical—your body—to express something spiritual. Exercise brings benefit to both body and spirit. Some forms, such as yoga, are especially well-suited for integrating the physical and the spiritual because they intentionally increase awareness of the difference that even small changes can make in fitness and stress reduction.

— DAILY HEALTH JOURNAL —

Number of steps .... ○ Add 3 servings of vegetables
○ Add 2,000 steps   ○ Add 3 glasses of water

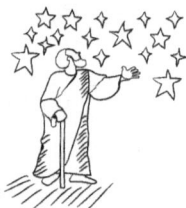

Week Two in Review

THIS WEEK WE HAVE READ about God's promise to Abraham, Abraham's questions about the impossibility, and the reassurance of God that the promise is true.

What promises have you made, to yourself or others, that you have not fulfilled? Perhaps you have made a promise to change a habit only to find that you gave up before you even started. It is human nature to fall short, but that is not God's nature. We learn the true meaning of a promise from God's ability to keep a promise, not from our inclination to break a promise.

If you struggled through some of your health goals this week, don't get discouraged or give up. Have patience and be grateful for a new chance to adjust your goals. Working on small changes consistently will lead to big changes over time.

Transfer your daily steps in the space below. If you set a goal for all three categories, put checkmarks in the boxes where you reached your goal for each day.

Number of steps	Add 2,000 steps	Add 3 vegetables	Add 3 glasses of water
Day 1	○	○	○
Day 2	○	○	○
Day 3	○	○	○
Day 4	○	○	○
Day 5	○	○	○
Day 6	○	○	○
Day 7	○	○	○

Keeping Promises

GENESIS 16:1-3

And Sarai said to Abram, "You see that the Lord has
prevented me from bearing children."
—Genesis 16:2

IMAGINE THE CONVERSATIONS Abram had with his wife, Sarai, about his encounters with God and the promise of too many offspring to count. They had no children, they were aging, and they had been living in Canaan for ten years. Yet Sarai was supposed to believe they would have an heir? Her patience wore thin, as ours also does when we don't see the results we hope for quickly enough. In Sarai's mind, it seems, God is not coming through on the promise. Besides, what Sarai did when she suggested that Abram take her servant as a wife and have a child with her was a culturally acceptable option. A child born to this union would be a legal heir.

If we're honest, we admit we recognize ourselves in Sarai. She got attached to the idea of something that was not happening and looked for what we would call a "workaround"—not ideal, but it gets the job done for now. It gives us what we want in the short term without addressing the core issue that causes the problem we're trying to solve.

When we look for shortcuts to better health, we misunderstand the wholeness that God wants us to experience. Health in body and spirit over a lifetime doesn't come from shortcuts but from patience and consistency and connection to God.

HEALTH TIP

It may take time for your efforts at exercise or healthy eating habits to make measurable differences in lower cholesterol, improved blood pressure, and increased energy. Respecting your body's rhythms and limitations requires humility, patience, trust, and perseverance. In the meantime, a health coach or exercise partner can be of great benefit. You don't have to go it alone.

— DAILY HEALTH JOURNAL —

Number of steps........................

⃝ Add 2,000 steps

⃝ Add 3 servings of vegetables

⃝ Add 3 glasses of water

Family Dispute

GENESIS 16:4-6

When [Hagar] saw that she had conceived,
she looked with contempt upon her mistress.
—Genesis 16:4

ALTHOUGH SHE GOT EXACTLY what she wanted—Abram's child in the womb of Hagar—Sarai came to regret her decision to give her servant to Abram. Everything backfired. When Hagar knew she was pregnant, the power shifted in her relationship with Sarai. Hagar had something Sarai believed she would never have, impending motherhood.

Now Sarai blamed the whole idea on Abram, who seemed to want to stay out of the conflict and told Sarai to handle it as she saw fit. Perhaps he did not foresee that Hagar would reach a point where being on her own with a child would be preferable to the way Sarai made a play to regain power by mistreating her. Hagar ran away. Now no one was getting what they wanted, and a child was at risk.

The choices of Abram, Sarai, and Hagar all make us flinch because they are familiar. While we may not have the complications of a polygamous culture, our household relationships remain complex. Family dynamics are not always emotionally healthy, and this contributes to behavioral choices that are not healthy, either. Multiple levels of ill health become a cycle.

If you recognize unhealthy cycles in your household, consider what steps are within your ability to improve relationships for the sake of everyone's health.

HEALTH TIP

One thing can lead to another. As in Sarai's case, a sequence of decisions can lead to unintended consequences. Bit by bit, our society has seen a gradual increase in food portion sizes. Even our plates are bigger, and soft drinks are at least 16 ounces. One step back toward balance is watching portion sizes. People lose significant amounts of weight simply by not eating any food portions larger than a fist.

— DAILY HEALTH JOURNAL —

Number of steps............................ ○ Add 3 servings of vegetables

○ Add 2,000 steps ○ Add 3 glasses of water

Running Away
GENESIS 16:7–9

*"Hagar, slave-girl of Sarai, where have you
come from and where are you going?"*
—**Genesis 16:8**

HAGAR'S HAUGHTINESS TOWARD Sarai once Hagar became pregnant with Abram's child was one factor in the household tension, and despite her slave-girl status, Hagar risked running away from Sarai. The angel of the Lord found her on the road to Shur, near Egypt. The angel knew who she was, calling her by name. Then the angel asked two questions—where have you come from and where are you going?—but Hagar answered only the first by referring to the emotional landscape of her home—"I am running away." While the road might take her to Egypt and she had Egyptian roots (Genesis 16:1), she did not seem to have specific intentions beyond getting away from Sarai.

If the angel had said, "Why? What did Sarai do to you?" Hagar no doubt would have had an answer. Instead, the angel said, "Return to your mistress, and submit to her." This was not what Hagar wanted to hear, and it may even sound harsh given Sarai's mistreatment of Hagar. But Hagar was alone, pregnant, and crossing the wilderness without a long-term plan because of rash decisions. The angel's words were a way of saying, "It's not too late to reconsider what is best."

We sometimes make emotional choices without accepting responsibility for circumstances or considering the consequences. We just want out! Hagar's encounter with the angel prods us to evaluate whether we make decisions in healthy ways.

HEALTH TIP

Children learn a lot about life from observing their parents. If parents exercise regularly and prepare nutritious meals, their children will learn healthy habits. The recommended amount of physical activity for children is about an hour a day to combat obesity. Some of this can come in the form of washing the dog, planting flowers, helping to clean the garage, or other activities that welcome the contributions children make to the household as well as build up their emotional health.

— DAILY HEALTH JOURNAL —

Number of steps.................................

○ Add 2,000 steps

○ Add 3 servings of vegetables

○ Add 3 glasses of water

DAY 18

Transforming Encounters

GENESIS 16:10-12

"You shall call him Ishmael, for the
LORD has given heed to your affliction."
—Genesis 16:11

HAGAR **DECIDED TO RUN AWAY** from Sarai, but the angel of the Lord told her to go back. Before Hagar could protest, the angel spoke a blessing to Hagar. God promised to multiply her offspring in the same way that God said Abram's descendants could not be counted. Hagar's child would be a son, and God chooses his name, Ishmael. This child's name means "God hears" and reassures Hagar that God knows her suffering and cares for her in the midst of it.

Despite God's plan to multiply Hagar's offspring, the son she carried would not be without faults or live an easy life. Often we think that if we can just fix the problem in front of us, everything will be all right. Life will get better. Our troubles will finally be behind us. Realistically, life is a mixture of peaceful, satisfying seasons and times of struggle and challenge.

The mixed-bag blessing that Hagar receives echoes the mixed-bag blessing Abram received in the promise of many descendants but the truth that they would be enslaved (Genesis 15:13–16). We should not confuse the word blessing with a belief that life will be free of troubles. Instead, a blessing reminds us of God's care and presence even in times of affliction.

HEALTH TIP

Until relatively recently, medical research has focused on men, and women have been under-represented in clinical trials. Women often receive diagnoses and treatment based on what has worked for men. For instance, heart attack symptoms in women may differ from those in men, leading to misdiagnosis. A broadened approach to research has begun to yield insights into the health-related similarities and differences between men and women. Take this into account when making an action plan for better health.

— DAILY HEALTH JOURNAL —

Number of steps............................   ○ Add 3 servings of vegetables

○ Add 2,000 steps   ○ Add 3 glasses of water

Sacred Spaces
GENESIS 16:13–16

"You are El-roi;" for she said, "Have I really seen
God and remained alive after seeing him?"
—Genesis 16:13

AFTER RECEIVING A BLESSING FROM God and the assurance that God sees her affliction, Hagar names God *El-roi*, meaning "God of seeing" or "God who sees."

Hagar was an Egyptian who perhaps joined the household of Abram and Sarai during their time in Egypt seeking relief from a widespread famine (Genesis 12:10–20). Although at first she tried to dodge the angel's questions (Genesis 16:8), she did not seem shocked that the Lord would seek her out to speak to her, so perhaps she was exposed to the faith story of Abram and Sarai while she served them. Now this foundation enables her to enter into her own transforming encounter with God and to recognize it for what it was. God saw her, promised to care for her, and restored her to purpose. In response, Hagar speaks words of gratitude and marks the experience as one that changed her.

The sacred place of this encounter, a well along the road, was called Beer-lanai-roi, which means "well of the Living One who sees me" or "well of the one who sees me and lives." Hagar is full of wonder and praise that God would initiate this encounter with her.

Hagar returned to Sarai and bore Abram's son, Ishmael. We learn from Hagar that when circumstances are so difficult that we want to escape, we can still find health-giving purpose and meaning in responding to God's call.

HEALTH TIP

Doctors know that giving a name to symptoms can help a patient. Counselors assist clients in naming their feelings. Parents put time and thought into choosing a name for a child. Simply naming barriers to good health can give us power over them. On the flip side, taking the time to reflect and name our health successes builds confidence for the next goal. Pause today and review the progress you've made, and then give it a name.

— DAILY HEALTH JOURNAL —

Number of steps............................ ◯ Add 3 servings of vegetables
◯ Add 2,000 steps ◯ Add 3 glasses of water

Abram's New Name

GENESIS 17:1–6

*"No longer shall your name be Abram,
but your name shall be Abraham."*
—**Genesis 17:5**

ABRAM WAS 75 WHEN GOD FIRST called him to journey to a strange land. He was 86 when Ishmael was born. And he was 99 when God appeared to him again to confirm the promise of offspring too numerous to count. This is the fourth time God appeared to Abram since he came into Canaan with essentially the same message (see 12:7, 13:14–17, and 15:1–6). This time God adds a new dimension to the encounter—changing Abram's name to one that embodies the covenant promise.

Abram means "exalted father." *Abraham* means "father of many." People of the Jewish and Christian faiths remember Abraham as the father of the Israelites, but through Ishmael he is also the father of Arab peoples. Through the children of Keturah, a future wife after Sarah's death, he is the father of still other people groups.

While Abraham lived most of his life with the name *Abram*, we remember him most as Abraham, whose faith God counted as righteousness despite the mistakes he made.

We all have a past. We all have experiences we wish we could have "do overs" for and make better choices. The greatness for which Abraham is remembered was still ahead of him when he was 99 years old. Don't believe that past failures and regrets must define your health in the future. Great things lie ahead.

HEALTH TIP

Many of us have a natural tendency to stay with what is familiar, and even habits that are not healthy are at least familiar. It takes courage and motivation to begin and sustain a healthy lifestyle. Abraham's new name conveyed a new image, but it took a long time for him to actually become "the father of multitudes." It may take a long time for efforts at forming new health habits to take root, but eventually they will begin to feel familiar and the old ways will seem as strange as Abraham's old name.

— DAILY HEALTH JOURNAL —

Number of steps................................ ○ Add 3 servings of vegetables

○ Add 2,000 steps ○ Add 3 glasses of water

Unto All Generations

GENESIS 17:7-8

"And I will give to you and to your offspring after you,
the land where you are now an alien."
—Genesis 17:8

GOD'S COMMITMENT TO the covenant with Abraham was forever. We have already heard God's promise four times, and there is more to come before Abraham's story is finished. God will give Abraham offspring and land, and his offspring will one day live in the same land where Abraham was a foreigner. In fact, the heart of the covenant is a theme that runs through the Old Testament, appearing in prophetic writings of Jeremiah, Ezekiel, Hosea, and Zechariah. Through Abraham, God's people are established, and biblical writers return again and again to the theme of God's care and protection.

But Abraham did not live for hundreds of years to see all this unfold, or to see how God would bring salvation into the world through Abraham's descendants. At this point in Abraham's story, he has been waiting 24 years for the beginning of the covenant promise—a son with Sarah. God asked Abraham to believe in a future promise and to imagine how the future might look, even though he could not see the future in the present moment.

This is the heart of hope: believing that the future can be different than the present swirling around us, and that we can participate in God's work of bringing good news into our lives and the lives of others. This is true in bodily health, relational health, emotional health, and spiritual health. God's promise is one of hope.

HEALTH TIP

As you reach the midpoint of walking with Abraham and Sarah, call on your faith and imagination to help you maintain enthusiasm to add 2,000 steps, add 3 servings of vegetables, and add 3 glasses of water each day. Take time to imagine how these lifestyle changes are leading you to improved health, happiness, and longevity. With hope, imagine a future full of the wholeness, love, and joy God wants you to experience.

— DAILY HEALTH JOURNAL —

Number of steps................................ ○ Add 3 servings of vegetables
○ Add 2,000 steps   ○ Add 3 glasses of water

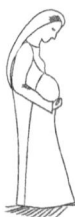

Week Three in Review

THE END OF THIS WEEK marks a milestone in the *Walking with Abraham and Sarah* program. Congratulations on reaching the halfway point!

Behavior changes require time and determination. The best way to break an undesirable habit is to replace it with a healthier habit, and it takes 21 days of practicing a new behavior to make it a habit. Even if you make mistakes along the way, try to see them as opportunities for growth rather than as failures that mean you will never succeed. If you have been easily meeting your goals, consider making them slightly more challenging for the remaining weeks of the program.

Surround yourself with supportive people who will lift you up when you fall down and motivate you to keep going. As you add steps to your day, you may discover new faces along your route. Maybe you already have discovered opportunities to talk with neighbors or an old friend. Perhaps you've had opportunities to swap stories with members of your congregation who are also making lifestyle changes. Your steps toward a healthier you are already bringing blessings into your life as you make new connections and work toward your goals.

*Transfer your daily steps in the space below. If you set a goal
for all three categories, put checkmarks in the boxes
where you reached your goal for each day.*

Number of steps	Add 2,000 steps	Add 3 vegetables	Add 3 glasses of water
Day 1	O	O	O
Day 2	O	O	O
Day 3	O	O	O
Day 4	O	O	O
Day 5	O	O	O
Day 6	O	O	O
Day 7	O	O	O

Outward Signs
GENESIS 17:9-13

"So shall my covenant be in your flesh an everlasting covenant."
—Genesis 17:13

G OD INSTRUCTED THE Hebrews to practice a sacred ritual that marked each male as a member of God's covenanted people. This physical act signified being consecrated to God and inheriting the promises that God made to Abraham for all of his descendants to come. Abraham was 99 years old when he received this sign, but in the thousands of years since, baby boys in the Jewish tradition have been circumcised when they are eight days old, as God instructed (Genesis 17:12). They bear in their bodies the mark of a distinct spiritual relationship between God and the covenanted people.

In later periods of Jewish history, leaders and prophets reminded the people to also think of circumcision of the heart. Physical circumcision was important, but it should not be separated from the spiritual understanding of belonging to God's people and being set apart to trust and serve God.

Many religious traditions, both ancient and contemporary, ask followers to adopt a "sign" of their commitment and belonging to the faith community. For instance, Christians are baptized as the mark of belonging to the faithful.

How do we mark ourselves as being faithful in our health journeys? We are not faithful simply because we develop the disciplines that are good for our bodies— nutrition and movement. We are faithful when we do these things because we understand they are part of the wholeness and abundant life that God intends for us to experience.

HEALTH TIP

Many of the Hebrew religious rituals had both spiritual significance and health benefits, such as the laws related to cleansing utensils and washing before eating. In the Jewish faith, circumcision is performed as a sacred ritual, but recent studies confirm that circumcision can also be a powerful weapon against transmission of HIV infections. The World Health Organization recommends voluntary male circumcision as part of AIDS prevention programs in regions with epidemic levels of infection.

— DAILY HEALTH JOURNAL —

Number of steps.................................   ○ Add 3 servings of vegetables
○ Add 2,000 steps   ○ Add 3 glasses of water

DAY 23

Sarai's New Name
GENESIS 17:15–16

"I will bless her, and moreover I will give you a son by her."
—Genesis 17:16

A FEW VERSES EARLIER WE SAW THAT GOD changed Abram's name to Abraham to reflect his role as the "father of many" in the covenant God established. Now his wife, Sarai, receives the name more familiar to us—Sarah. Both forms of her name mean "princess," but in renaming her, God specified that she would be the mother of nations and kings. The blessing God offered to Abraham extended to his wife. Thus she had her own role to play in God's covenant people.

God promised Abraham descendants as uncountable as the stars. Then came the time that Sarah tried to move the promise along by giving Hagar to Abraham to have a son with her. Now God makes clear that the promised offspring would begin with a child Sarah would bear. By now Abraham was 99 and Sarah was 89. They began this journey with God almost a quarter of a century earlier.

If we put ourselves in Abraham's shoes at this moment, we might think, "Those are lovely words, but they must be metaphorical. If what you said was impossible 25 years ago, it is even more impossible now." This can be a sign of discouragement, and we begin to settle for less than what God wants to give us. If you begin to feel this way, remind yourself that God really does want to you to be healthy in both body and spirit.

HEALTH TIP

Expectant mothers need to be especially attentive to nutrient guidelines and should avoid alcohol and smoking during pregnancy. But there are times when both men and women who are otherwise healthy may need supplemental vitamins, minerals, and nutrition. A good example is the need for extra calcium and vitamin D for all women after menopause to help prevent osteoporosis, which puts women at additional risk of bone fractures.

— **DAILY HEALTH JOURNAL** —

Number of steps........................   ○ Add 3 servings of vegetables
○ Add 2,000 steps   ○ Add 3 glasses of water

Great Doubt

GENESIS 17:17–19

Then Abraham fell on his face and laughed.
—Genesis 17:17

CAN WE BLAME ABRAHAM? He fell down laughing at the suggestion—even from God—that Sarah would have a son. He did the simple math: current ages plus one year, to allow time for a pregnancy, would make them parents at 100 and 90 years of age. Perhaps he even fell on his face in order to hide his laughter. But he had the good sense to keep these thoughts to himself. Instead he said aloud, "O that Ishmael might live in your sight!" Perhaps God could be redirected to a more sensible solution. Ishmael was a young teenager by now, living as the only son in a wealthy household. In a few more years there would be reason to believe grandchildren would begin to come.

But there was nothing metaphorical about God's words. God immediately redirected Abraham to the promise that Sarah would bear a son. This child, not Ishmael, would inherit the covenant promises. God even told Abraham the child's name—Isaac, which means "he laughs."

We are not so different from Abraham. When we are caught in a moment of disbelief, we may laugh at the absurdity or try to rearrange the elements in a way that makes more sense. This happens even in our choices about issues that affect our health. We benefit when we stay on the topic that God establishes for us rather than trying to readjust truth in our own ways.

HEALTH TIP

Like Abraham, when we don't know how to respond, sometimes we laugh. But sometimes we laugh because something is genuinely funny—and it's good for us. Laughter provides a physical and emotional release and can even decrease stress, increase pain tolerance, and support the immune system. What makes you laugh? A favorite television show? A witty friend? Humorous stories? Find the people who will laugh with you and see how much better you feel.

— DAILY HEALTH JOURNAL —

Number of steps................................ ○ Add 3 servings of vegetables
○ Add 2,000 steps ○ Add 3 glasses of water

DAY 25

This Season Next Year
GENESIS 17:20-22

"But my covenant I will establish with Isaac,
whom Sarah shall bear to you at this season next year."
—Genesis 17:21

GOD HAS NOT FORGOTTEN ISHMAEL. God promised blessing to Ishmael before the boy was born and will keep the promise. Ishmael will become the father of 12 sons and ultimately a great nation. But the covenant God made with Abraham would continue through Isaac, the son yet to be born. In one more year, the long wait to truly understand the promise God made so many times for Abraham's descendants would come to fruition. As impossible as it sounded, in one more year, Abraham and Sarah would hold a son in their arms.

Perhaps by now Abraham stopped believing God was serious, and God had the last word. "And when he had finished talking with him, God went up from Abraham" (Genesis 17:22). The encounter was complete.

Abraham waited a long time for this moment. Now it was up to him to decide how he would respond to everything that had just happened. We all have moments in our pursuit of health when information or insight comes to us and then it is up to us to respond with positive action.

HEALTH TIP

Abraham had to wait one day at a time for the birth of Sarah's son. Health comes one day at a time. When larger goals feel impossible, we can support our health habits by saying, "Just for today I will take care of my body," "Just for today I will exercise my spirit," "Just for today I will love myself and others." Write down one or two "just for today" sentences that will encourage you to stay on track with positive action.

— DAILY HEALTH JOURNAL —

Number of steps.................................   ◯ Add 3 servings of vegetables

◯ Add 2,000 steps   ◯ Add 3 glasses of water

Following Instructions
GENESIS 17:23-26

*Abraham was ninety-nine years old when
he was circumcised in the flesh.*
—Genesis 17:24

DESPITE BEING STUNNED AT GOD'S assurance than he and Sarah would have a son in a year's time, Abraham took prompt and positive action to do what God had instructed. He followed through on making sure that all the men in his household—himself, Ishmael, and servants and slaves who would have been numerous in a wealthy household—were circumcised. Though he could not see generations ahead to what the covenant promises ultimately would mean, Abraham attended to the goal that was right in front of him.

Many cultures today practice circumcision out of a conviction that it brings health and hygienic benefits. In some places, boys are circumcised as infants, while in others circumcision is a rite of passage when boys approach puberty. Similar practices were common in the Near East in the ancient time of Abraham.

It was not that Abraham had never heard of circumcision before. The difference was that his obedience of God's command established a covenant community. Generations later, Moses repeated the command that male infants should be circumcised on the eighth day because the rite welcomed the children into the covenant promises that God made to Abraham.

A place of belonging is essential to human health and thriving. Where are the communities where you belong, feel supported, and have the opportunity to make a contribution?

HEALTH TIP

Aside from its religious symbolism, circumcision has long been debated in medical circles. Every operation, at any age, has risks and benefits. Before making a decision about a procedure, become informed. In the age of the Internet, many of us go first to this vast source of information. It is important to identify trustworthy Internet sites that present information based on research, not opinion. If you have questions about what you read, ask your physician.

— DAILY HEALTH JOURNAL —

Number of steps.................................. O Add 3 servings of vegetables
O Add 2,000 steps   O Add 3 glasses of water

DAY 27

The Welcome Mat

GENESIS 18:1-8

[Abraham] said, "My lord, if I find favor with you,
do not pass by your servant."
—Genesis 18:3

IN THIS PASSAGE, WE READ GOD'S fifth appearance to Abraham since the journey began nearly 25 years ago. The Lord appeared with two angel companions both to reiterate that Sarah would have a child (Genesis 18:10) and warn Abraham that disaster was coming to Sodom, where his nephew Lot lived (Genesis 18:20–21).

Hospitality under the circumstances was common in the ancient Near East. The harsh climate, vast arid areas, scarcity of water, and the uncertainty of accommodations meant that hospitality could make the difference in surviving the journey. In the summers, temperatures in the Negeb, where Abraham lived, could reach 110 degrees. Travelers would seek relief from the heat of the day, and residents would gladly offer it. Water, bread, shade—all this would be a normal exchange.

Yet Abraham seemed to recognize that these were not ordinary travelers. Perhaps this is what prompted him—at age 99—to hurry to greet them. He involved his wife, not merely servants, in the food preparation and offered far more than bread and water. While the visitors ate, Abraham stood nearby ready to serve them in any way that might arise.

Hospitality is a gift. We offer a sense of welcome and care. This glimpse of Abraham's response to visitors reminds us that we also can recognize and welcome the ways God comes to us, which may be in the form of unexpected guests or in the faces of strangers.

HEALTH TIP

Our experience of travel is very different than in the days of Abraham, but we still can be challenged. When you travel, think ahead to how you can continue to support your health goals while away from your normal routine. Make sure to pack medications and a pair of comfortable walking shoes. And smile at people you meet. Such a simple act of welcoming people into your experience will bring benefit to you and to them.

— DAILY HEALTH JOURNAL —

Number of steps............................   ○ Add 3 servings of vegetables
○ Add 2,000 steps   ○ Add 3 glasses of water

Startling News
GENESIS 18:9–15

"Is anything too wonderful for the LORD?"
—Genesis 18:14

I N THIS VERSION OF THE LORD PROMISING a son to Abraham and Sarah, we see Sarah's view up close for the first time. Sarah was listening from inside the tent to her husband's conversation with the three visitors. Imagine when she heard them talking about her! Perhaps Abraham had already told her about his last meeting with God, in which the time frame of one year was revealed, and perhaps she had laughed then as well. Certainly she laughed now, with the same doubt that Abraham had expressed. They are advanced in age. It is ridiculous to even allow themselves to consider that the outlandish might come true.

Now imagine Sarah's expression when she heard the Lord say to Abraham, "Why did Sarah laugh?" Quickly she tried to cover her tracks with fear cloaked in denial. "I did not laugh." God simply said, "Oh yes, you did laugh." God knows the doubt we carry in our hearts and the ways we shut ourselves off from the goodness God offers.

Sarah was left to savor the words, "Is anything too wonderful for the Lord?" Being caught in her untruth did not mean she was any less confused about how this promise would be fulfilled. Even when we want to believe the impossible could happen, we still wrestle with how. Yet moments of confusion are opportunities to open our eyes in faith and remember that God does indeed keep promises.

HEALTH TIP
It is common to relate healthy lifestyles to our bodies, but healthful living integrates the spirit as well. Your spirit needs attention during busy times, with the chance to relax and connect to deeper matters than the next thing that needs doing. One of the best antidotes for modern-day busyness is the practice of Sabbath. When was the last time you slowed down and treated your body and spirit to a day of leisure and restoration?

– DAILY HEALTH JOURNAL –

Number of steps........................   O Add 3 servings of vegetables
O Add 2,000 steps   O Add 3 glasses of water

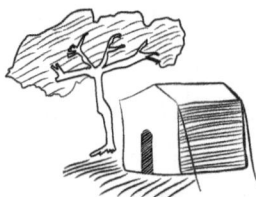

Week Four in Review

IT'S INTERESTING THAT THE FINAL Scripture reading this week dealt with age and health. Like Sarah, many of us may feel like we are much too old to do certain things. Too old to dance. Too old to play sports. Too old to change our habits.

When we get up in years, we find it acceptable to assume our aches and pains are associated with age. The truth is most of us will benefit by doing more activities as we get older. If we continue to stay active and incorporate movement into every day, we retain more muscle mass and range of motion in our joints. In our 20s and 30s, losing range of motion seems unimaginable. But when in our 40s and 50s we find ourselves having difficulty with what used to be simple tasks, we might have more understanding of how someone who is 60 or 70 feels.

No matter what age you are now, it is never too late to change a habit. Patience, tolerance, perseverance, and a sense of humor will all help you stay focused on your healthy habits.

Transfer your daily steps in the space below. If you set a goal for all three categories, put checkmarks in the boxes where you reached your goal for each day.

Number of steps	Add 2,000 steps	Add 3 vegetables	Add 3 glasses of water
Day 1	O	O	O
Day 2	O	O	O
Day 3	O	O	O
Day 4	O	O	O
Day 5	O	O	O
Day 6	O	O	O
Day 7	O	O	O

Backsliding

GENESIS 20:1-8

*While residing in Gerar as an alien, Abraham said
of his wife Sarah, "She is my sister."*
—Genesis 20:2–3

"**S**HE IS MY SISTER." **DOES THAT LINE** sound familiar? Once again Abraham was in a new place and suspected his wife may attract attention, so he relied on an old lie to ease the transition. We might think Abraham should know better. Didn't he learn his lesson well the first time, when years earlier he told the pharaoh in Egypt that Sarah was his sister (Genesis 12:11–13)?

Perhaps one of Sarah's appealing qualities was belonging to a wealthy household. Abimelech, a local king, might have been looking to both increase his wealth and establish an alliance by taking Abraham's "sister" into his household.

"Don't do this," God said to Abimelech, holding him back from making things worse. Abimelech defended his innocence: he did not know Sarah was married, and he had not touched her. Then he learned that God was not there in judgment but in grace. It was God who restrained Abimelech and who simply instructed Abimelech to return Sarah to her husband.

Why did Abraham choose the lie? Perhaps he thought he was doing what would best protect all the people he was responsible for. What would happen to them if he was killed? But God was again gracious, even in the way he spoke of Abraham to Abimelech: "he is a prophet and he will pray for you" (Genesis 20:7). God remained gracious, and this is a truth for all of us to hang onto.

HEALTH TIP

We all slip up. We eat those brownies we were determined to avoid at the office party or skip exercise so many times that we lose momentum. We neglect important relationships or over-schedule ourselves to the point of fatigue. Remember that God is gracious, and be gracious to yourself. One mistake, or making the same mistake more than once, does not permanently derail forming new health habits. Start again, and seek support from others to help you stay on track.

— DAILY HEALTH JOURNAL —

Number of steps ....   ○ Add 3 servings of vegetables
○ Add 2,000 steps   ○ Add 3 glasses of water

Caught!

GENESIS 20:9-13

And Abimelech said to Abraham,
"What were you thinking of, that you did this thing?"
—**Genesis 20:10**

ABRAHAM, FOR HIS OWN REASONS, put Abimelech in a situation where he made one regrettable decision and very nearly made things worse. Now Abimelech demanded an explanation: "What were you thinking?" Abraham admitted what he was thinking, even if it was misguided. First he acted on an assumption that turned out to be wrong—that there was no fear of God in Gerar, where Abimelech ruled. He assumed a hostile environment where he did not expect to experience God's presence or provision. So we have this glimpse into Abraham's decision making and perhaps see a bit of ourselves in it. We find ourselves in stressful situations and do whatever it takes.

But then Abraham tried to fall back on the technicality that Sarah was his half-sister, so technically he had not lied to Abimelech. In fact, although we see just two instances of Abraham and Sarah using this scheme, verse 13 ("at every place") indicates that it was an ongoing plan for the last 25 years.

We're not so different from Abraham. Most of us have some sort of backup plan for when things don't go well and are ready to take matters into our own hands and justify our choices later. The better choice is not to assume that God will not be present and gracious when we face difficult situations.

HEALTH TIP

Can self-examination be a health practice? Yes. When we are tempted to do what is expedient rather than what is best, as Abraham was, a few deep breaths can help us slow down and think more clearly before we act. What will bring meaning and satisfaction into our lives in the long run? If we pause to examine our motivations and desires, we will be more likely to make choices that nurture positive relationships and sustain healthy habits.

--- **DAILY HEALTH JOURNAL** ---

Number of steps............................ ○ Add 3 servings of vegetables

○ Add 2,000 steps ○ Add 3 glasses of water

Making Things Right
GENESIS 20:14–18
Abimelech said, "My land is before you;
settle where it pleases you."
—**Genesis 20:15**

ABIMELECH TOOK SARAH INTO HIS household presumably to become one of his wives, a custom that would not have been unusual for a king in ancient times. God came to Abimelech to stop his actions. Abimelech pleaded innocence because he did not know Sarah was Abraham's wife and immediately went back to Abraham to straighten things out.

Even though the complex situation began not in Abimelech's wrongdoing but in Abraham's deceit, Abimelech now went over and above to bring restoration. Rather than extending his own wealth and prestige through bringing Sarah into his household, he increased Abraham's wealth with livestock, slaves, and silver. As he returned Sarah to her husband, he made clear that she was exonerated from any suggestion of wrongdoing.

Then Abraham did what God told Abimelech he would do; he prayed for Abimelech. Verse 17 tells us "God healed Abimelech" along with the women in his household who had been temporarily infertile while Sarah was there. In an age and culture that put heavy value on having many children, this mattered a great deal. Abraham and Sarah knew this well, having been childless for the length of their marriage.

However this muddle began, it closes with a picture of mercy and restoration and healing. When we get in over our heads and make choices that affect our health for emotional reasons or as coping strategies, we can remember that wholeness is still the direction where God leads us.

HEALTH TIP
Forgiveness is a concept that flows off the pages of the Bible from beginning to end. We forgive others because God forgives us. Forgiveness is a great example of the connection between body and spirit. Forgiving those who hurt us, even deeply, brings multiple health benefits, such as lower blood pressure, better sleep, improved energy, and even a longer lifespan. If you are holding onto hurt, it might be harming your health. What would it take for you to let go?

– DAILY HEALTH JOURNAL –

Number of steps............................. O Add 3 servings of vegetables
O Add 2,000 steps O Add 3 glasses of water

DAY 32

A Boy Named Laughter

GENESIS 21:1-8

"Who would have ever said to Abraham that Sarah would nurse children? Yet I have born him a son in his old age."
—Genesis 21:7

WHEN THE THREE VISITORS CAME TO ABRAHAM and Sarah and told them they would have a son in another year—at ages 100 and 90—they both laughed. We see a humorous side of God when God tells Abraham that the child's name will be Isaac—meaning "he is laughing."

Abraham and Sarah's laughter at the prediction of a son's birth was the type that comes from nerves, disbelief, or doubt. But God did as promised, and a year later Sarah held a little boy in her arms. In Isaac's name, *laughter* took on the happier meaning of expressing joy and celebration.

Remembering the covenant that God made with Abraham, and the promise that Sarah's son, rather than Hagar's, would be the son of the covenant, Abraham obeyed God's instructions and circumcised his newborn son. As Abraham and Sarah watched their son grow, his name would also be a daily reminder that God kept the promise despite the years they grew tired of waiting or the times they were tempted to take things into their own hands.

Most of us have people or objects in our lives that remind us of a past season that may have been difficult. Those same people or objects can also be reminders that God is faithful, and remembering that encourages us in the journey toward wholeness.

HEALTH TIP

Studies suggest that women over 35 face special risks during pregnancy and delivery. For example, women over 35 are twice as likely as younger women to develop high blood pressure and diabetes for the first time during pregnancy. The risk of a child having a chromosomal disorder increases as a woman ages, as do rates of miscarriage and placental problems. Most woman over 35 can look forward to normal pregnancies and healthy babies, but it's especially important to obtain prenatal care.

— DAILY HEALTH JOURNAL —

Number of steps............................   ○ Add 3 servings of vegetables
○ Add 2,000 steps   ○ Add 3 glasses of water

Painful Parting

GENESIS 21:9-20

*The matter was very distressing to
Abraham on account of his son.*
—Genesis 21:11

WHEN HAGAR WAS PREGNANT, Sarah exerted her power. Hagar ran away.

God sent Hagar back, and Ishmael was born (Genesis 16). Thirteen years passed before the three visitors told Sarah her son would be born in another year. After Isaac arrived, the two sons, a toddler and a teenager, lived in the same household.

We know nothing about Hagar and Sarah's relationship in the intervening years, but now Sarah's emotions reared up again. She didn't like the sight of Ishmael playing with his young brother and asked Abraham to send Hagar and Ishmael away (Genesis 21:9–10). While 16 or 17 years ago Abraham had been willing to let Sarah mistreat Hagar and seemed passive in the story, this time he has difficulty with the thought of sending away his nearly grown son. God repeated the promise that Ishmael would become a great nation, so Abraham gave Hagar some provisions and sent her away.

When Hagar ran out of water in the wilderness and was desperate, God came to her, repeated the promise to make her son a great nation, and opened her eyes to a well. We see more of Ishmael many years later in the book of Genesis, so we know God preserved him, just as God promised

Physical thirst also serves as a reminder of spiritual thirst for God, especially in times of distress. Where along your journey does God show you unexpected refreshing wells?

HEALTH TIP

Water is a substance of life! Our bodies are two-thirds water. We do not have to become as desperate as Hagar was in the wilderness before recognizing how much our bodies need water. One of the easiest steps to take for better health is simply to drink more water. Start with replacing just one beverage a day with a glass of water. Then aim for 64 ounces or more of water each day.

— DAILY HEALTH JOURNAL —

Number of steps.................................   O Add 3 servings of vegetables
O Add 2,000 steps   O Add 3 glasses of water

DAY 34

An Unimaginable Instruction
GENESIS 22:1-3

[The Lord] said, "Take your son, your only son Isaac, whom you love, and go to the land of Moriah and offer him there as a burnt offering."
—Genesis 22:2

MORE YEARS HAVE PASSED. Isaac is no longer a toddler and was perhaps a teenager himself when God tested Abraham. We flinch at the idea of being tested by God, especially when God asked Abraham to sacrifice something as precious as the son God had so clearly promised and given him. Sarah is not in this scene, but it is not difficult to imagine what her reaction must have been if Abraham told her where he was going and why.

Reading this part of the story, we sense a climax is coming. Abraham's life has certainly been dramatic, yet once again when God called him he answered, "Here I am." And he did not dillydally or put off obedience with excuses. The next verse tells us Abraham got up early, loaded the donkeys, took Isaac and two servants, and left.

What must have been going through his mind? What faith it must have taken to believe that even in these circumstances God would bring good. Our own faith journeys—and health journeys—have climax moments when we must step out in faith that God will bring good no matter how impossible the circumstances feel.

HEALTH TIP

We hesitate to talk about nutrition because we're afraid we might be asked to sacrifice favorite foods. However, like Abraham, we could be in for a surprise. Nutritionists can find delicious alternatives or advise how much of a favorite food we may indulge in. For example, fat is often considered a "bad" food, but in fact ten percent of our total caloric intake should be poly- or monounsaturated fat. The more we know about nutrition, the more choices we have.

— DAILY HEALTH JOURNAL —

Number of steps................................   ○ Add 3 servings of vegetables
○ Add 2,000 steps   ○ Add 3 glasses of water

Faith in a Crisis

GENESIS 22:3–10

"We will worship, and then we will come back to you."
—Genesis 22:4

For Abraham, obedience to God required a lot! God told him to sacrifice his son Isaac, the child of the promise. He traveled for several days. Abraham had cut wood for the burnt offering before he left home, so his son and servants would have known he intended to make a sacrifice. But Abraham alone carried the weight of knowing what God asked of him. Did he speak during those days? Try to distract himself? Pray? By the third day, the sacrifice site was still some distance away, but at this point Abraham left the servants behind.

Notice what he said. "We will worship, and then *we* will come back." This is a statement of great faith that even if he followed through and sacrificed his son, somehow God would restore Isaac to him and the two of them would return to the servants.

So often we want to look ahead and see the end of things. What *exactly* is going to happen? What *exactly* is God going to do? Abraham did not know the answer to these questions, yet he moved forward into the next stage of the journey. His faithfulness is an example to us even as we go step by step on the road to health. God asks for our faithfulness in each moment, not only when we can be sure we like the end of the story.

HEALTH TIP

We get to a better state of health in stages. We can't take shortcuts, we can't hope for a miracle drug, we can't see a preview of the end of the story. We may become disillusioned if we don't get weight loss or fitness results in the short term. Combining movement with proper nutrition will bring slow and steady results that can be sustained.

— DAILY HEALTH JOURNAL —

Number of steps.........................   ○ Add 3 servings of vegetables
○ Add 2,000 steps   ○ Add 3 glasses of water

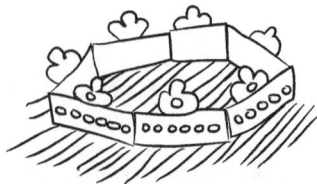

Week Five in Review

WE HAVE NOW COMPLETED FIVE weeks of *Walking with Abraham and Sarah*. Take some time to take stock not only of the progress toward your goals but also what other benefits have come out of these weeks. One benefit may be that you have built connections with other people who are also walking with Abraham and Sarah. Whether you followed along with one other person as you monitored your activity or were supported by many, having people around to cheer you on and take an interest in your progress improves results and makes the journey more enjoyable.

Look to your supporters to stay focused on your journey. Think how much more difficult many of the decisions Abraham faced would have been without Sarah by his side. In some moments we are strong and able to be the moving force for co-pilgrims. In other moments, need to let someone lead and strengthen us. We all benefit from knowing that we are not alone. This week take time to thank God for the people who support your efforts and let them know how much you appreciate them.

Transfer your daily steps in the space below. If you set a goal for all three categories, put checkmarks in the boxes where you reached your goal for each day.

Number of steps	Add 2,000 steps	Add 3 vegetables	Add 3 glasses of water
Day 1	○	○	○
Day 2	○	○	○
Day 3	○	○	○
Day 4	○	○	○
Day 5	○	○	○
Day 6	○	○	○
Day 7	○	○	○

The Lord Will Provide

GENESIS 22:11–14

So Abraham called that place
"The Lord will provide."
—Genesis 22:14

A BRAHAM BOUND HIS SON AND laid him on the wood. Thinking of what this was like for Isaac gives us shivers—especially after his father had assured him that God would provide the lamb for the offering (Genesis 22:8). Now his father raised the knife with purpose.

Did Abraham hesitate? Did his hand shake? Did tears stream down his face?

Abraham went right up to the edge of his faith—and that is where God showed up, calling his name twice. "Here I am," Abraham said, perhaps with his knife still raised. God commended Abraham for his faith and told him not to touch his son. The heart-pounding moment was over. Abraham looked up and saw a ram caught in the thicket. This was to be the sacrifice, not Isaac.

Abraham held nothing back. This was what God asks of us—to follow wholeheartedly. Even when things do not make sense. Even when things are gutwrenchingly hard. Even when we hope and pray another solution will come. Abraham called that place, "The Lord will provide," a label that we, too, can carry into the difficult moments when abundance feels far away.

Most of us are more comfortable when in control of the circumstances of our lives. May we open our minds and hearts to a deeper trust in God's provision in those seasons when God asks for our obedience.

HEALTH TIP

Both faith and healthy lifestyles are integral to the whole person. Sometimes, though, we can be tempted to substitute words of faith for the action of healthy choices. Prayer helps to guide and assist us in making and implementing our choices, but faith is not meant to take the place of our actions toward maintaining health.

— DAILY HEALTH JOURNAL —

Number of steps...........................

O Add 2,000 steps

O Add 3 servings of vegetables

O Add 3 glasses of water

DAY 37

The Nations Are Blessed
GENESIS 22:15–19

"Because you have done this, and have not withheld your son,
your only son, I will indeed bless you."
—**Genesis 22:16–17**

AGAIN AND AGAIN GOD SHOWED faithfulness in Abraham's life. In various circumstances, and at various times over the span of years, God repeated the promise to give Abraham and Sarah a lasting legacy through their descendants. Once before, in Genesis 15:5, God used the image of offspring as numerous as the stars, and this is again the picture God speaks to Abraham. To underscore and multiply the impact, God also says Abraham's descendants will be like the sand on the shore. And not only will Abraham's family be blessed through the promise, but "all the nations of the world" will be blessed (Genesis 22:18). Ultimately this promise was fulfilled by God's Son coming into the world through Abraham's line.

Both stars and sand are pictures of the vastness of what is possible with God. This all rises from Abraham's obedience. We have seen occasions when Abraham's faith wavered and when he made choices that did not have health and wholeness at the heart of them. But Abraham has drawn closer to God and strong in faith, and because of that Christ's healing presence came into the world.

God took one person, Abraham, and promised blessings to more people than Abraham could count. Sometimes we think what we do doesn't matter in the long run. But when we offer our obedience, even in the way we live out our understanding of health, God can do great things.

HEALTH TIP

Companionship on the health journey makes a difference! Community is a wonderful way to multiply blessing by sharing stories, offering encouragement, and celebrating successes. Look around. Who are the people with whom you can share and receive God's blessing in ways that support health and wholeness? You don't have to plan a massive program or time commitment; just look for small ways to show you're thinking of companions on the way and notice the difference it makes for you and others.

— DAILY HEALTH JOURNAL —

Number of steps ....   ○ Add 3 servings of vegetables
○ Add 2,000 steps   ○ Add 3 glasses of water

A Funeral

GENESIS 23:1-4, 17-20

After this, Abraham buried Sarah his wife in
the cave of the field of Machpelah facing Mamre.
—Genesis 23:19

N OW THE STORY OF ABRAHAM and Sarah fast-forwards to the death of Sarah, who lived another 37 years after the birth of Isaac and saw her longed-for son grow into adulthood and become a grown heir for Abraham.

Even after all his years of living in Canaan and gaining prosperity, Abraham saw himself as a foreigner who needed to seek out a place to bury his wife. He bought a field with a cave, and there he buried Sarah on land that faced Mamre, where the three visitors had come to tell Abraham and Sarah that Isaac would soon be in their arms.

This is the first mention we have of Abraham owning a part of the land he has been living on all these years. He lived in tents and moved around. But now, with the death of his wife, he owns a piece of the land that God promised to him and begins a new season of legacy for his family. Abraham did not want to bury Sarah on borrowed land but in a place where he could also one day be buried.

Families build legacies, whether intentionally or unintentionally. Abraham's legacy was Isaac, the son of the promise, and now a piece of the promised land. Both the son and the land reflect his true legacy of faith in God not just in a moment of crisis but over the span of his life.

HEALTH TIP

Most families have traditions that are passed on from one generation to the next. Make sure you are passing on healthy habits to children, grandchildren, or other extended family members. Move together. Prepare healthy food together. Talk about significant events together. Be sad together and glad together. Personal example is a powerful legacy for health and wellness, so live a positive example.

─ **DAILY HEALTH JOURNAL** ─

Number of steps................................   O Add 3 servings of vegetables
O Add 2,000 steps   O Add 3 glasses of water

A Proposal
GENESIS 24:1-18

"Go to my country and to my kindred
and get a wife for my son Isaac."
—Genesis 24:4

I N ABRAHAM'S TIME MARRYING WITHIN the extended family was preferred. This kept the family name, property, and possessions within the tribe, and this is behind the urgency Abraham expressed that Isaac must marry within Abraham's family. His oldest servant, who had "charge of all that he had," was now entrusted with the most important decision about Isaac's future and Abraham's legacy. But Abraham and Sarah had left their own country long ago, and they had no family around them. The servant would have to travel to the homeland to find a bride.

This was no small feat. The bride must be from Abraham's family, her own parents must support the marriage, she herself must be willing to leave the life she knew to marry a man she had never met. Yet Abraham speaks with confidence that the servant will be successful because God will be present in the arrangements.

Abraham's faith in the promise was contagious. When the servant arrived in the family's homeland, he prayed for God to bring the right woman to him. Abraham and Sarah initially received God's promise, and now we see the servant demonstrating faith and participating in its fulfillment. What happens to us, and how we respond to circumstances, affects those around us. In this picture of how the faith of Abraham spilled over into other lives, we find encouragement to use our faith to support the health and wellness of those around us.

HEALTH TIP

Just as Abraham's faith led to faith in others—for generations—abundance in our understanding of health flows from one small seed that begins the process. Making healthy lifestyle changes to benefit both body and spirit means putting down roots in our commitment to new habits and watering the seed with nutrition, exercise, work, and relationships that welcome others into the journey.

— DAILY HEALTH JOURNAL —

Number of steps ....   ○ Add 3 servings of vegetables

○ Add 2,000 steps   ○ Add 3 glasses of water

An Engagement
GENESIS 24:50–42, 55–59

*"Do not delay me, since the LORD has
made my journey successful."*
—Genesis 24:56

ABRAHAM SENT A TRUSTED SERVANT to find a wife for his son Isaac. Before the servant had even finished praying beside a well for God's guidance in identifying the right woman, he met Rebekah, the daughter of Bethuel, the son of Abraham's brother Nahor and his wife Milcah. God confirmed the choice when Rebekah did just was the servant asked for as a sign—offered to draw water from the well for the camels.

After receiving expensive gifts from a stranger, Rebekah must have suspected the encounter held great meaning. Her family agreed to the arranged marriage, but hesitated about sending Rebekah off with the servant as immediately as he wished. They wanted more time to adjust to the change—just ten days. But the servant was eager to let Abraham know the mission had been successful and pressed for an immediate departure. The decision came down to Rebekah. She would be leaving everything she knew. How quickly was she prepared to make this transition?

Rebekah was ready. And despite not having a few more days with Rebekah, her family sent her off with a blessing that echoes God's promise to Abraham of myriad offspring. Riding on a camel, Rebekah traveled toward a future she did not yet know but on which she had fixed her sight.

HEALTH TIP

Sometimes breaking away from what is familiar helps us to grow. At times like this we muster our spiritual, emotional, and physical resources to move into the unknown. Making lifestyle changes is one of those challenges. Decreasing unhealthy habits and increasing healthy habits is not always easy, but maintaining a vision of the future we are moving toward will help us take each new needed step.

— DAILY HEALTH JOURNAL —

Number of steps ....   O Add 3 servings of vegetables
O Add 2,000 steps   O Add 3 glasses of water

A Wedding
GENESIS 24:62-67

He took Rebekah, and she became his wife; and he loved her.
—Genesis 24:66

ABRAHAM AND ISAAC COULD HAVE had no quick way to get word that the servant had been successful and that Rebekah was on her way. Isaac was still mourning his mother's death (Genesis 24:67) while also anticipating his own future.

Most marriages at the time were not based on love, and in fact romantic love was not one of the requirements Abraham held for the marriage of his son. Yet the writer of Genesis gives us a glimpse of the affection that quickly grew between Isaac and Rebekah. He was out for an evening walk when he caught her eye for the first time. When she realized this was her intended husband, she fastened the customary veil of an unmarried woman across her face.

The servant told Isaac everything that happened. Isaac must have been raptly listening to the account of how God had led the servant to the right woman to bring back to marry Isaac. Perhaps this story of God's provision contributed to how quickly Isaac loved his new wife. The chapter ends with the note that his marriage brought him comfort after the loss of his mother. We don't forget the people we lose, but often other events or relationships that happen after the loss help us to see that it is possible to enjoy a life of healing and wholeness in the mercy and provision God continues to offer to us.

HEALTH TIP

Grief is a painful process we are tempted to avoid. But ignoring feelings of loss and sadness can be unhealthy and may lead to stagnation, listlessness, and depression. The grieving process is different for everyone. The common thread is completing these four steps: accepting the loss, dealing with physical and emotional pain, adjusting to life without the person lost, and moving on. We don't have to forget a loved one in order to find a "new normal" that moves us forward.

— DAILY HEALTH JOURNAL —

Number of steps............................ ○ Add 3 servings of vegetables
○ Add 2,000 steps   ○ Add 3 glasses of water

The Death of Abraham
GENESIS 25:1–10

His sons Isaac and Ishmael buried him the cave of Machpelah ...
There Abraham was buried, with his wife Sarah.
—**Genesis 25:9–10**

ABRAHAM LIVED FOR SOME TIME AFTER Sarah died and had another wife (or concubine) named Ketura, who bore him six more sons. He provided for all his sons, but Isaac remained the son of the promise who inherited Abraham's estate. Abraham lived to be 175 years old, which means Isaac, at 75, was no longer a young man himself. Abraham's death was an occasion for the return of Ishmael, who was in his late 80s. We do not know any details of the relationship between Abraham's sons in the years since Sarah asked Abraham to send Hagar and Ishmael away, but the end of the story is that they buried their father together.

Funerals can be difficult times, with emotions on edge and grief sometimes lowering our ability to speak kindly and patiently, or to set aside the kinds of grudges that happen in complicated households. This story reminds us first of all that Abraham lived to a "good old age" and "full of years." He had a long, fulfilling life worthy of celebrating. Then it reminds us that two children who had grown up under a shadow were both, as mature adults, able to come together to pay their last respects. Even stressful times can carry aspects of healing when we open ourselves to the possibility.

HEALTH TIP

A number of studies confirm the positive correlation between spirituality and improved health and quality of life, especially among the elderly and terminally ill. Many health care providers leave the spiritual realm to ministers, but surveys show that many patients would like health care workers to include the spiritual dimension of healing in their care, and they respond positively when this happens. An integrated approach satisfies the need for all aspects of the patient to be embraced in the healing process.

— DAILY HEALTH JOURNAL —

Number of steps.........................
○ Add 2,000 steps

○ Add 3 servings of vegetables
○ Add 3 glasses of water

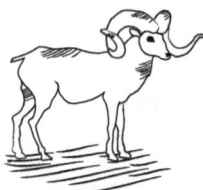

Week Six in Review

AS WE FINISH SIX WEEKS OF *Walking with Abraham and Sarah*, we reflect on the lives of past generations and how those generations are a piece of who we are today. From great ancestors we never knew, who lived thousands of years before us, to those we remember from just a generation ago, all of them leave footprints in our hearts.

Have you thought about the footprints you leave for future generations? How will you be remembered? How would you like to be remembered? Sometimes we are remembered for the little things we do, phrases we use, or the way we laugh. And sometimes we are remembered for a family tradition we began or passed down. We can also be remembered by the way we live our lives with healthy habits and our pursuit of love and joy in a life close to God.

Thinking about the past six weeks of *Walking with Abraham and Sarah*, how are the goals you set fitting into your lifestyle? Are there choices you made during the program that you hope to continue? Your health decisions can have an impact on others, ultimately influencing your family, friends, congregation, and wider community.

Transfer your daily steps in the space below. If you set a goal
for all three categories, put checkmarks in the boxes
where you reached your goal for each day.

Number of steps	Add 2,000 steps	Add 3 vegetables	Add 3 glasses of water
Day 1	O	O	O
Day 2	O	O	O
Day 3	O	O	O
Day 4	O	O	O
Day 5	O	O	O
Day 6	O	O	O
Day 7	O	O	O

— Congratulations! —

YOU HAVE COMPLETED *Walking with Abraham and Sarah*. By increasing your steps, adding 3 servings of vegetables, and adding 3 glasses of water each day, you have taken some steps in the right direction.

It's important to continue the lifestyle changes you've made during the last six weeks. Treat yourself to a new pair of walking shoes. Explore a museum, zoo, or nature preserve. You may even consider walking in a charity 5K with a friend. Think of fun ways to reward yourself that will relate to your new lifestyle and motivate you to continue your new habits.

Please take a few minutes to answer the following questions and return the completed form to your project coordinator.

Name: ....

Congregation or Community Organization: ....

1. I was able to add 2,000 steps to my daily activity.
   ○ Never   ○ Seldom   ○ Sometimes   ○ Often   ○ Always

2. I was able to add 3 servings of vegetables to my daily meals.
   ○ Never   ○ Seldom   ○ Sometimes   ○ Often   ○ Always

3. I was able to add 3 glasses of water to my fluid fluids.
   ○ Never   ○ Seldom   ○ Sometimes   ○ Often   ○ Always

4. I found *Walking with Abraham and Sarah* to be helpful and it inspired me to reach my goals.
   ○ Never   ○ Seldom   ○ Sometimes   ○ Often   ○ Always

5. How many days a week do you engage in some type of mild to moderate physical activity (walking slowly, gardening, housework, window shopping, and so on)?   **Days per week** ....

6. How many days a week do you engage in some type of moderate to vigorous physical activity (brisk walking, running, riding a bike, dancing, playing a sport and so on)?   **Days per week** ....

CUT HERE

7. Which answer best describes how you feel about the following?

	I have no plans to	I plan to in the future	I plan to immediately	I have been doing so for *fewer* than six months	I have been doing so for *more* than six months
Increasing physical activity					
Improving nutrition					

8. To what degree do you feel that your physical health and spiritual health are connected?

○ Not at all   ○ Quite a bit

○ A little bit   ○ Extremely

○ Moderately

9. What comments would you like to share with the project coordinator?

Thank you for participating! Please return this form to the project coordinator in your congregation or community organization.

CUT HERE

CONTINUE THE JOURNEY TO HEALTH

More from the Ways to Wellness series ...

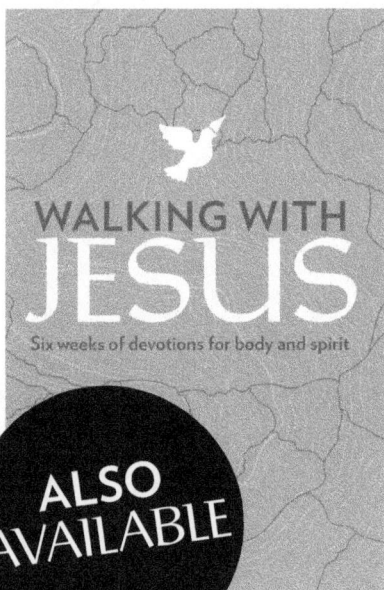

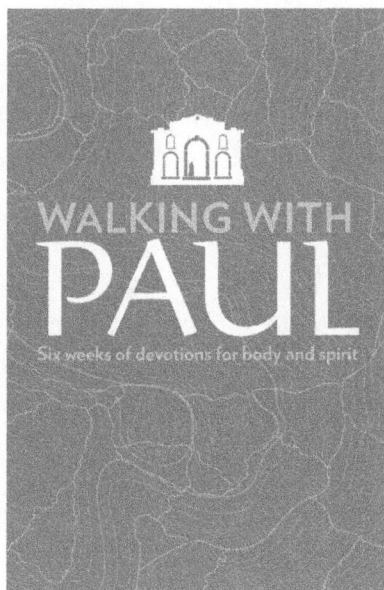

Work on health goals for six weeks
while meditating on Scripture readings
that follow the walking routes of
JESUS and **PAUL**.

About the Author

SUSAN MARTINS MILLER has been a writer and editor for over 30 years, creating faith-based resources for children and adults to use both at home and in congregational settings. She holds a master's degree in biblical studies (New Testament) from Trinity Evangelical Divinity School.

Walking with Abraham and Sarah is part of the Ways to Wellness series, which also includes *Walking with Jesus* and *Walking with Paul*.